The Thinking Man's 12-WEEK Guide to Gaining SIZE

By R. Conrad Bingham, D.D.S., NASM-CPT

WARNING!

> The high intensity routines in this book are intended for health
> men and women. People with health problems should not
> attempt these routines without a physician's approval. Before
> beginning any exercise or nutrition program, always consult
> your doctor.

DEDICATION

I dedicate this book to my Lord and Savior, Jesus Christ, my wife, and three children, who have supported and inspired me to become all that I can be.

CONTENTS

INTRODUCTION

The bodybuilder's goals are to get bigger, have incredible muscle size, awe-inspiring arms and chest, massive thighs, and bigger, stronger body parts.

Few bodybuilders, however, reach their goals. Most fall short because they stray from the fundamentals. In their pursuit for massive muscles, they superset, and bombard, rotate and split, and amino acid their bodies into a deep state of overtraining. They train too much, load their bodies with excessive protein, and rest too little.

In short, the vast majority of bodybuilders fail to acquire the results they disparately want. More or less, they don't get any bigger.

The 12-week program I'm about to lead you through is established on one of the oldest, time-tested methods for gaining strength and muscle. This type of training has successfully prepared just about every type of athlete conceivable, from Olympic weightlifters to soccer players. It works so well that it has been practiced continually for decades. I myself have tried out some unusual exercises and combinations, but occasionally you have to rely on the basics. That's especially true when a basic program works as well as this one. Of course, I have taken this basic, but really effective program and fine-tuned it to perfect its effectiveness and to maximize the results you get. These results include greater strength, bigger muscles, lower body fat and a more "cut-up" body.

So, why is it that even with all the training, and excess protein and little rest, bodybuilders frequently have trouble getting bigger? It's because of acclimatization.

These are forms of adjustment to environmental stresses, which are usually reversible, whether they occur in childhood or adulthood.

The different forms of Acclimatization are long-term, seasonal, and short-term, in terms of the amount of time it takes for the change to occur. Tanning is a common form of seasonal acclimatization

An example of a long-term acclimatization is people who lose excess body fat and are very slender as a result of mild, long-term undernourishment. If they later increase their diet to a consistent level of excessive calories, they will very likely retain more body fat and in time, become obese. They experience long-term acclimatization when they initially lose body fat and again later when they retain it. In both cases, they are acclimatizing to the available food supply.

Anatomical and/or physiological adjustments also may develop over even shorter time periods. For example, a lot of people acquire dark skin tans during the summer months and lose them during the wintertime. This modification in skin coloration is a seasonal acclimatization to the damaging consequences by ultraviolet radiation from the sun.

When skin divers descend into the ocean, they experience rapidly increased water pressure within seconds, they can suffer from agonizing pain in their ears due to the unequal pressure inside and outside of their eardrums. They must equalize this pressure by blowing hard through their nose. By doing this, they are making a short-term acclimatization to the changed environment. Changing water pressure necessitates short-term acclimatization for skin divers.

The difference between the kinds of acclimatization is not only in the amount of time it takes for the accommodation to initially happen. Usually, the shorter the time for acclimatization, the faster it is also in reversing once the environmental stress is no longer present.

Developmental adjustment doesn't only result in defects and disorders. Dietary alterations as well, can have a positive effect if nutrition is improved. This has been the case in Japan since the end of World War II. The Japanese Education Ministry on January 31, 1996, reported that children have been significantly taller in each generation since then. In 1986, for instance, 14-15 year old Japanese boys averaged 7 inches taller than did corresponding aged boys in 1959. A key changing factor in Japanese lifestyle has been diet. It's likely that this was by and large responsible for the increased body size. Between 1961 and 1971, Japanese consumption of animal protein rose 37% while plant food consumption dropped 3%. In the cities of Japan and other increasingly affluent areas of East Asia, food habits have changed dramatically over the last several decades. Hamburgers, pizza, fried chicken, and other high fat Western foods are very popular with the young and affluent. In Japan today about one fourth of the calories consumed are fat--this is 5 times higher than just after WWII. Lending support to the hypothesis that diet changes of this sort can result in significant developmental adjustments is a recent two year study of children in Kenya. It found that the inclusion of only 60 grams (about two spoonfuls) of meat a day to the diet of young children resulted in the development of 80% greater upper-arm muscle compared to children who were rigid vegetarians. A diet that included a comparable amount of milk instead of meat resulted in an increase of 40%. Foods of animal origin are important in the diet of young children because they contain nutrients that are hard to obtain from non-meat or non-dairy sources. However, too much animal protein and fat can result in obesity and other health hazards.

Exercise training is an adaptive process. The body will accommodate to the stress of exercise with increased fitness if the stress is above a minimum threshold intensity. To achieve maximal effectiveness, we must consider factors involved in the adaptation of muscle to stress and deconditioning. These factors include overload, specificity, reversibility, and individual differences.

An interesting aspect of skeletal muscle is its adaptability. If a muscle is stressed (within tolerable limits), it adapts and improves its function. For example, weight lifters exercise their arms and shoulders, so their muscles hypertrophy and improve their strength. Larger muscles allow them to adapt to an increased load. Similarly, if a muscle receives less stress than it's used to, it atrophies. For example, the muscles of a casted leg atrophy in response to disuse.

The purpose of physical training is to stress systematically the body so it improves its capacity to exercise. Physical training is beneficial only as long as it pushes the body to adapt to the stress of physical effort. If the stress is not adequate to overload the body, then no adaptation occurs. If a stress cannot be tolerated, then injury or over-training results. Significant advances in performance come about when the appropriate exercise stresses are introduced into the athlete's training program. Physical fitness is for the most part, a reflection of the level of training. When an athlete is working hard, fitness is high. However, when heavy training discontinues, fitness commences to deteriorate.

There are innumerable exercise devices and training programs available that are heralded as the most effective way to gain strength. In most instances, as long as a threshold tension is developed, increases in strength will come about. The type of strength developed is the important consideration in exercise and sports. Long distance running up steep hills, for example, will produce a certain amount of muscular strength. The muscular adaptations that result will differ from those produced from high resistance, low repetition squats (knee bends). The distance runner develops mainly sarcoplasmic protein (oxidative enzymes, mitochondrial mass, etc.), while the weight lifter develops primarily contractile protein. The nature of the adaptive response must always be considered when designing the training program.

Factors That Determine Rate and Type of Strength

The factors that determine the rate and type of strength gains include overload, specificity, and reversibility.

Overload

Muscles increase their strength and size when they are forced to contract at tensions close to their maximum. Muscles must be overloaded to hypertrophy and improve strength. Experimental and empirical observations have allowed generalizations concerning the amount of overload necessary for strength gains.

Muscle protein accumulation occurs by increasing the rate of protein synthesis, decreasing the rate of protein degradation, or both. Fiber types differ in their response to overload. Slow fibers hypertrophy by decreasing the rate of protein degradation. Fast fibers hypertrophy by increasing the rate of protein synthesis. The rate of protein synthesis in a muscle is directly related to the rate of entry of amino acids into the cells. Amino acid transport into muscle is influenced straight off by the intensity and duration of muscle tension. This was determined by experiments with isolated muscle. They were bathed in a solution containing labeled amino acids, such as 14C labeled a-amino isobutyric acid. It was found that amino acid uptake was highest when muscles were contracted. Uptake was greater as tension and the duration of tension increased.

Weight training studies and empirical observations of athletes have reinforced the importance of generating muscular tension. It must be developed at an adequate intensity and duration for the optimal development of strength. The majority of studies have found that the ideal number of repetitions are between four and eight (repetitions maximum, 4-8 RM). They should be practiced in multiple sets (3 or more). Strength gains are less when either fewer or greater numbers of repetitions are used. These findings are consistent with the progressive resistance training practices of athletes.

Athletes involved in speed-strength sports practice low repetition, high intensity exercise during or immediately preceding the competitive season. These athletes include shot-putters and discus throwers. Such training improves explosive strength, while allowing sufficient energy reserves for practicing motor skills. However, the effectiveness of this practice has not been established experimentally.

Body builders usually do more sets and repetitions of exercises and more exercises per body part than weight lifters or strength athletes. Their goal is to build large, defined, symmetrical muscles. It is not known if typical body building training method is the most effective means of achieving their goals. Numerous studies have shown that high resistance, low repetition exercises are more effective than low resistance, high repetition exercises in promoting muscle hypertrophy.

Proper rest intervals are crucial for maximizing tension, both between exercises and training sessions. Insufficient rest results in poor recovery and a diminished capability of the muscle to exert full force. Unfortunately, the ideal rest interval between exercises has not been determined. Most athlete's strength train three to four days per week with large muscle exercises, such as the squat and bench press, rarely done more than twice a week. This practice has been empirically derived. It allows adequate recovery between training sessions.

The overload must be progressively increased for consistent gains in strength to occur. However, because of the high risks of over-training in strength building exercises, perpetually increasing the resistance is sometimes counter-productive. A relatively new practice among strength trained athletes is periodization of training. This practice alters the volume and intensity of exercises so the nature of the exercise accentuate frequently changes. Many athletes think that this practice produces a faster rate of adaptation. Periodization of training will be discussed further in the section on the progressive resistance training programs of athletes.

Specificity

Muscles adapt specifically to the nature of the exercise stress. The progressive resistance training program should stress the muscles how they are to perform. The most obvious example of specificity is that the muscle exercised is the muscle that adapts to training. Thus, if you exercise the leg muscles, they hypertrophy rather than the muscles of the shoulders.

There is specific recruitment of motor units within a muscle depending upon the requirements of the contraction. The different muscle fiber types have characteristic contractile properties. The slow twitch fibers are relatively fatigue-resistant, but have a lower tension capacity than the fast twitch fibers. The fast twitch fibers can contract more rapidly and forcefully, but they also fatigue rapidly.

The use of a motor unit is dependent on the threshold levels of its alpha motor neuron. The low threshold, slow twitch fibers are recruited for low intensity activities such as jogging (and for that matter, most tasks of human motion). However, for high speed or high intensity activities, such as weight lifting, the fast twitch motor units are recruited.

The amount of training that occurs in a muscle fiber is determined by the extent that it is recruited. High repetition, low intensity exercise, such as distance running, uses mainly slow twitch fibers. Endurance training improves the fibers' oxidative capacity. Low repetition, high intensity activity, such as weight training, causes hypertrophy of fast twitch fibers. There are some changes to the lower threshold slow twitch fibers. The training program should be structured to produce the desired training effect.

Increases in strength are very specific to the type of exercise, even when the same muscle groups are used. Specific motor units are recruited for specific tasks. If a person is weight training to improve strength for another activity, the exercises should be as close as possible to desired movements. Likewise, when attempting to increase strength after an injury or surgery, rehabilitation should include muscle movements as close as possible to normal activities.

 Muscle fiber type appears to play an important role in determining success in some sports. Successful distance runners have a high proportion of slow twitch muscles (percent slow twitch fibers is highly related to maximum oxygen consumption). Sprinters have a predominance of fast twitch muscles. Several studies have shown that a high content of fast twitch fibers is a prerequisite for success in progressive resistance training. This is understandable, as the fast twitch fibers experience selective hypertrophy as a result of high resistance, low repetition exercise.

However, all sports do not require prerequisite fiber characteristics. For example, in world class shot-putters there is a surprisingly diverse muscle fiber composition. In those athletes, larger muscle fibers rather than percent fiber type, accounted for their performance. There are differences in the relative percentage of fast twitch fibers in explosive strength athletes. Having a high percentage of fast-twitch fibers is not necessary critical for success. Many strength athletes have a higher fast-to-slow twitch fiber area ratio than in sedentary subjects and endurance athletes. Individual differences in training intensity and technique can make up for deficiencies in the relative percentage of fast twitch fibers in these athletes. It would be interesting to speculate about the performance of a shot-putter with a high percentage of fast twitch fibers. What would performance be like in an athlete who developed good strength and technique? The high percentage of fast twitch fibers would probably be a decided advantage.

Simultaneous participation in a training program designed to stimulate both strength and endurance has been found to interfere with gains in strength. Strength athletes may inhibit their ability to gain strength by participating in vigorous endurance activities. Muscles may be unable to adapt optimally to both forms of exercise.

Reversibility

Muscles will atrophy as a result of disuse, immobilization, and starvation. Muscles adapt to increasing levels of stress by increasing their function. Disuse leads to decreasing strength and muscle mass. Atrophy results in a decrease in both contractile and sarcoplasmic protein.

The muscle fiber types do not atrophy at the same rate. Joint immobilization results in a faster rate of atrophy for the slow twitch muscle. This has important implications for rehabilitation. Often, increasing strength is a major goal following immobilization. Endurance should also be stressed because of the relatively greater loss of slow twitch muscle capacity.

Immobilization affects muscle length. If a muscle is fixed in a lengthened position, sarcomeres are added, while they are lost if the muscle is immobilized in a shortened position. Immobilization also leads to a variety of biochemical changes including decreased glycogen, adenosine diphosphate (ADP), creatine phosphate (CP), and creatine. All of these factors can affect muscular performance after immobilization has ended.

Individual Differences

As with other forms of exercise, people vary in the rate they gain strength. Some of these differences can be attributed to the relative predominance of fast- and slow-twitch motor units in muscles. Usually, endurance athletes will have more slow twitch fibers (Type I motor units) in their active muscles. Strength athletes will have more fast twitch fibers. Intense progressive resistance training mainly enlarges fast-twitch fibers. People who have more fast-twitch fibers will tend to gain strength faster than those who do not.

Muscle strength is related to the cross-sectional area of the muscle. However, this strong relationship diminishes when "explosive athletes" and endurance athletes are compared. What most studies suggest is that strength is highly related to muscle size. However, people who have a disproportionate amount of fast-twitch fibers will gain strength faster than those who do not. Fast-twitch fibers tend to be stronger than other fiber types, so people who have more of them will tend to be stronger and have greater potential for strength gains.

Several studies have shown that fiber composition is genetically determined. Genetic researchers often investigate the influence of heritability on a trait by studying monozygotic and dizygotic twins (identical and non-identical twins). Fiber distribution and muscle enzyme activity in monozygotic twins is almost identical in most of these studies.

Genetics is not the sole determinant of individual differences in strength. Numerous studies have shown that many successful strength-speed athletes do not have a predominance of fast-twitch motor units in critical muscles. Further, in athletic subjects, fiber composition is only marginally related to the time subjects can maintain isometric force and perform explosive squat jumps. Genetics exert a strong influence on the ability to gain strength. A good training program can make up for "genetic deficiencies."

Applying Basic Principles of Exercise Training

Adaptation is the whole purpose of exercise training. Adaptation requires a systematic application of exercise stress. The stress should be sufficient to stimulate an adaptation, but not so severe that breakdown and injury occur.

After a certain period of time, increases in size and strength ceases due to lack of sufficient stimulation to trigger continuing muscle adaptation. The muscles have basically finished accomplishing their goal of becoming big and strong enough to handle the resistance that they are placed under. This is the way the body handles stress.

The stress coping mechanism was termed the General Adaptation Syndrome by Dr. Hans Selye. When the body goes through repeated stress like high-intensity weight training, it encounters three levels of response:

1. **Alarm**. The period when the body adjust defenses as it prepares to compensate for the new stress.

2. **Resistance**. The body actually adapting to the stress by getting bigger

3. **Exhaustion**. Your body hits a wall, or plateau, and your gains are stalled as a state of overtraining sets in.

The 9 Signs You Have Hit a Plateau in Your Training

1. A Loss in Strength

A common sign of hitting a plateau or even beginning to enter the overtraining stage is when you suddenly experience a loss in overall strength.

Now I am not simply referring to when you don't progress in a workout or exercise. No. What I am talking about is when you notice a significant decrease in your performance and you can no longer match the lifts you once did.

This is a sign that your body has not been able to properly recover and grow more muscle tissue. Worst part is, sometimes, when you damage your muscles to this point, you become weaker. Hence this is why a loss in strength will occur.

2. Failure to Achieve a Pump

Although I do not believe achieving a pump when you are working out directly translates to muscle growth, I do believe that if you can no longer feel a pump in your muscles when you are working out that this is a sign that your body is not fully recovered.

Ever notice when you take a break from training, or when you first began working out, your muscles would fill up and you would get that famous 'pump' feeling?

Did you also notice you don't get that nearly as much the longer you have been training without a break?
This is yet another sign that you're on the road to overtraining which will inevitably lead to a plateau.

3. Lack of Motivation

When you lose motivation, it could be caused by a number of reasons such as personal matters, pursuit of different interests but if those are not your reasons then it is more than likely caused by hitting a plateau otherwise known as overtraining.

At this point, your body is tired, fatigued and doesn't feel like going to train with heavy weights. This is pure instinct and your body will tell your brain 'we need to recover...STOP training'.

You see, your body knows better than you might think. As a motivated trainer, you would more than likely just want to push through and try to blast through the plateau. Of course, in this case, you need to do the opposite. Hard to do I know, but you have to do this in order to let your body recover properly.

4. No Progress in At Least 2 Workouts

A good rule of thumb when trying to build muscle is to constantly progress in your workouts and exercises every week. The progression doesn't have to be much, but it does have to be enough to trigger new growth. This could be an extra couple of reps on your bench press or even adding 5% extra weight to your bench press and completing the same reps as you did previously with a lighter weight.

All these little progressions lead to new muscle formation through the 'adapt and grow' principle. When you are training hard, eating ample amounts of calories to build muscle and paying attention to recovery, you should have no problem progressing in your workouts.

However, if there comes a time when you have not progressed in any exercises of 2 consecutive identical workouts, then this should be a big sign that your body has reached a plateau and it's time for a change.

This rule only applies when you haven't progressed in ANY form. If you are having a hard time on just one exercise, but progressing in the other exercises of your workout, you are still progressing. You may just need to change the exercise you're having a hard time with.

5. **Feeling Flush**

This happens quite a bit amongst aggressive trainers. Feeling flush in the face is an indication of overworking your body past the point of comfort. It can be brought on by many different factors, but generally speaking, when you feel red in the face or your ears feel like they are burning, this could be a sign of overtraining or being over-stressed from numerous causes (work, training, emotionally).

It doesn't matter which is the primary cause, there is only one solution; rest and relaxation. Even if you know the cause is something going on in your personal life that's not related to training, it will still have an effect on your training.

Stress causes an increase in blood pressure which will in turn cause your face to become pink/red and flushed. Your body is smart, and it will give you the signs when it feels like you're not listening to it, and this is just another one.

For those of you, who have never experienced this, don't think that you are never overworked or stressed because that's not the case. You may just be the exception to the rule or your body might have a different way of signaling overtraining and stress.

6. Lack of Aggression and Increase in Irritability

Typically when you start to feel grouchy, down, slightly depressed or just don't have that same edge you first had when you started training, it may be a sign that you need to rest up and take a break from the gym.

Our bodies release large amounts of cortisol when we are stressed out and we can become stressed when we overwork our bodies. Cortisol works directly against any muscle building you might be trying to accomplish.

Generally when I don't have that same aggression factor when I am lifting in the gym, I know I am either on the verge or have already entered into a plateau.

What's the point of continuing to try and training at 50% of your regular intensity? You won't be setting any new personal bests when you are in this state, so the best thing to do is to take some time off and let yourself recover.

If you're just having a bad day and that's the reason behind your bad attitude, then don't worry, it happens. But, if this is consistent over several workouts, it may be a sign to cool it for a while.

7. No Progress in Muscle Gain in At Least 2 Weeks

If you are on a path to gain muscle mass, you should be aiming to gain about 1-2 lbs. per week. This is a good progression for lean muscle gain, and of course you can gain at a more accelerated rate if you're ok with a bit more fat gain.

Now if after one week, you don't gain anything on the scale, don't freak out just yet. After all, it happens and the best thing to do is simply look back on your past week or so of training, nutrition and rest. There are many things you can try, which I will cover later on, that will automatically get you back on track to gaining more muscle.

But if after two consecutive weeks, you don't see any increase in muscle mass or even weight, then chances are you have hit a plateau and will need to make some changes.

8. Variances in Resting Heart Rate

Although this might be a more advanced overtraining syndrome for some, it is still worth noting. Basically, there are two different types of overtraining syndromes that can affect your resting heart rate.

The Sympathetic Form: Common in physical activities such as sprinting or fast explosive heavy lifting.

The Parasympathetic Form: This form is more common in endurance type of activities such as higher rep training or long cardio sessions.

Both forms will have different effects on the resting heart rate and its fluctuations, but one thing is certain and that is overall performance suffers and fatigue sets in faster during exercise once you enter either of these two overtraining syndromes.

Sympathetic Form Effects on Resting Heart Rate: When one enters into the sympathetic form of overtraining, the resting heart rate can be excessively high when compared to your previous normal heart rate for a given activity. Basically, your heart rate will rise much higher than normal when in this state.

Parasympathetic Form Effects on Resting Heart Rate: When one enters into the parasympathetic form of overtraining, you might find it hard to sustain the same workout at the usual set point that you normally would. Your heart rate will be significantly decreased and you will more than likely fatigue prematurely without ever reaching the desired intensity or physical exertion you were aiming for.

In basic sense, you won't be able to match your normal heart rate even if exercising at the same intensity as before.

9. **Decrease in Appetite**

When things are going well in your training and you are eating clean and seeing good gains, you are typically hungry and can keep that appetite all day long.

But, when you begin to fatigue and you no longer have that aggressive edge when lifting, you might also notice a decrease in appetite. This is due to the fact that when our bodies become overworked and stressed, our muscle receptor sites can become 'tired' and are no longer as responsive to accepting those calories and shuttling into the muscles as stored glycogen.

At this point, your metabolism might feel sluggish and this is simply because a tired body is less efficient at everything it does which also includes nutrient assimilation, digestion and proper partitioning. All point to a sign of a potential plateau.

The Periodization Concept

This program is based on the training concept called periodization. Periodization is the method of changing up your training at specified time points. The very first periodized scheme to be used with weights is called Linear Periodization (also known as Classic Periodization). That simply means that you start guaranteed with light weight and high reps and as the program progresses the weights used get heavier and heavier and the reps completed per set get fewer and fewer. Most periodized programs take many months complete. Many last anywhere from 4 to 12 months to complete the cycle. But this periodized program utilizes a concept known as microcycles. Where a typical linear periodization scheme might stick with the same weight and rep range for a month or longer, the micro cycles change up the weight and rep ranges every week.

The constant increase in weight and reps for two weeks, then the dropping of the weight with slower reps, and the recycling of 2 phases, for 12 weeks, leads to impressive strength gains. The microcycles also lead to muscle hypertrophy due to the constant changing up of the rep ranges each and every week. Another reason for the strength and mass gains has to do with the fact that you keep the weight steady in each exercise for all sets and you're forced to complete the minimum number of reps in that range.

Greater gains in strength and muscle mass are guaranteed with this program. Impressive results with this program have been observed, in both men and women. There have been incredible gains of strength on squat and bench press, and increase in muscle mass. Some guys have gained over 15 pounds of muscle. Yes, pure muscle while, actually dropping body fat. Speaking of body fat, when maximizing body fat with my training and diet tweaks. Some men have lost over 20 pounds of body fat and women have also seen impressive gains in strength and muscle while losing body fat women following my program have increased their squat strength by over 60 pounds and bench press strength by 30 pounds and gains in muscle over 10 pounds and fat loss over 10 pounds.

But I'm not the only one reporting insane gains in muscle mass and size with con committed losses in body fat.

The first exercises you do for each muscle group, except for abs and calves, will remain constant through all 12 weeks. This is the exercise that you are focused on increasing your strength. Most of the assistance exercises that followed the first exercise will change every phase. For abs, the exercises will change each week, based upon the rep ranges. This is due to the fact that some abdominal exercises are easier to do for high reps, and are somewhat difficult to do for lower reps, so the best abs exercises were arranged for the prescribed rep ranges.

TIME TO GET FOCUSED.

As already mentioned, this program works well to increase the three main goals that we all have, increased muscle strength boosting muscle size and enhancing fat loss. To boost muscle mass as much as possible, we will be using high intensity techniques, rest pause, and drop sets.

Focus: maximizing muscle growth - during weeks 1 and 2 of each phase of the program, you will do one rest pause on the last set of each exercise to do this reach muscle failure on the last set direct the weight and rest for 15 seconds. Then continue the set until you reach muscle failure again. During weeks 3 and 4 of all phases you will do drop sets on the last set of each exercise. To do this, take the last set to muscle failure and immediately reduce the weight to the amount you used for the exercise during week one and continue the set until failure again.

As far as workouts go, the plan to do only weightlifting during the heavy phase-no aerobics. Lift as much weight as possible, to hit the lowest number of reps for that particular week. Using as much weight as possible, incorporate a deep stretch into the movement. Hit the eccentric (negative) hard, especially during the second week of each heavy phase. Rest a full three minutes between sets, in order to recover strength and to be able to lift heavy.

 It is important to stretch the connective tissue around muscle cells as much as possible while bulking up. Do this by stretching between exercises and actually doing as much stretching as I can during exercises. For example, on the lat pulldown and the low-pulley row, really stretching out the lats. On exercises like the dumbbell triceps extension, lower the weight as far as you can behind my head and really extend those muscles, and on exercises like the dumbbell preacher curl, extend the biceps muscles and stretch them out, all the way.

During the cutting phase, four days a week you're going to try to do a minimum of 20 minutes (but hopefully as much as 30 or 40 minutes) of aerobic exercise, on an empty stomach, to accelerate fat loss. After a workout, wait about an hour before you eat (your body will continue to burn fat for fuel at an accelerated rate after exercise). By then, you'll probably have to eat-you'll be starving.

During this phase, you're going to train with weights, doing moderate weight, relatively high reps, and relatively low intensity.

Your goal during this two-week period is to get rid of body fat while maintaining muscle mass. This phase is not about stretching the connective tissue or gaining muscle, so you're not going to exaggerate the stretching components on my exercises, nor are you going to work very hard on the eccentric reps. This is not the time for beating up your muscles-protein synthesis will probably be down during this phase, and recovery will be difficult.

Throughout the program, you're going to drink ample amounts of water-at least 80 to 100 oz. a day.

The Goal: Get Bigger!

Your goal is to put on three or four pounds of bodyweight during the heavy phase which sounds like a lot, considering if you've been training for many years. In theory, if you do everything right, two-thirds of the weight you gain should be lean mass.

During the cutting phase, you're going to try to lose all of the fat mass you gained during the bulking phase, while hopefully retaining most of the muscle. Then, you're going to immediately go back on another bulking phase. The second bulking cycle, after your body has been "primed" by a strict one-week dieting period, is when it really hits you-you notice your muscles getting drastically bigger and stronger. You'll love looking forward to that!

The Theory Behind Cycling Your Diet

Human beings have not evolved much during the last 100,000 years; thus, we are still developed for our hunter/gatherer and, more recently, pastoral ancestors, who, whenever they succeeded in killing an animal, lived on meat for a week or two. At other times, when they had misfortune hunting and a crop failed, they lived on a low-calorie diet. This selective pressure gave man adipose tissue with just about unlimited storage capacity and a very adaptive metabolism to deal with periods of different diets. So, that's what we're created for!

During a period of restriction, the body is optimized for a forthcoming period of "excess" consumption of calories. When this period takes place, the body will store excess calories at an enormous rate.

Therefore, if your goal is to not appear like an average person, you have to "trick" the body perpetually in order to grow.

By combining these two states-by cycling your calorie intake over the correct period of time, your average fat mass will not increase, but your average lean body mass will go up significantly!

The secret to my system is a two-steps forward, one-step back calorie cycling. You overfeed the body for only one week and then diet for one week.

Eating as much as the body's metabolism requires each day increases calorie intake considerably, that is a stimulus for muscle growth-even in adults. It's somewhat of a widely accepted fallacy that when you eat too much, whether it's hamburgers, donuts, or even healthy foods like fruits, vegetables, lean meats, etc., your body's only storage compartment for these excess calories is adipose tissue [fat].
  The truth is, overfeeding your body is actually more anabolic [causes more muscle growth] than training with weights! Unfortunately, overfeeding also produces an undesirable increase in fat mass, which is opposed to what most bodybuilders seek-they work to construct a lean, muscular physique, not simply one that takes up more space.

The trick is to somehow discovering a way to not increase bodyfat stores significantly. The secret is acute calorie cycling.

As long as you drastically increase calories, then reduce calories during each cycle, the body has to respond the way it is programmed to.

The long standing theory is throughout the evolution of man, there have always been times of plenty followed by periods of shortage.

Even though our ancestors had to be strong enough to fight and hunt, if they built too much muscle, their metabolic rates would get too high, and in the "old, old days," people with very high metabolic rates did not survive famines. Thus, the body adjusts, so after two weeks of overfeeding, the body becomes more efficient at storing excess calories in adipose cells.

 Basically what I'm saying here is that we have a small time window, really about 14 days-long. This is enough for muscle hypertrophy to occur, while short enough to keep a significant amount of fat from being stored in the adipose tissue. However, I'm recommending only one week. Many people find it challenging to shed two weeks of a high calorie diet.

 It's really quite fascinating when you think about it, and it's a logical theory. Can this be substantiated with rock-hard scientific data? No, not yet, but the available scientific literature offers evidence this is the way the human body works.

It flat out works. During the one-week heavy phase, you can eat just about anything you want, which is actually fun-guilt-free "junk food! If you begin an overfeeding program after a diet, within a matter of days, you'll notice an increase in muscle fullness and strength. It's absolutely "drug like" the way your body changes so rapidly.

The dieting phase is fairly hard, but similar to carb depletion, in preparation for a contest. The restriction of calorie intake for just two weeks is nothing equated to what many bodybuilders do-starving themselves for two, three, or even four months to get ready for a photo shoot or contest. Every time I get hungry, I always know it will be only a matter of days before I can eat just about anything I want again. This helps compliance a great deal.

During my dieting phases, I have been able to lose virtually all of the fat I gained on my bulking cycles while dropping only a couple pounds of lean mass. You might think of this program as a two-steps-forward, one-step-back program.

I have a number of "gym cronies" who I've had experimenting with the system, and their results have been very similar to mine. On each cycle, you'll gain between two and five pounds of muscle, which, for someone who has been training for over a decade, like I have, is a phenomenal thing to experience.

First of all, let's backtrack a bit and go over why it's so important to have a low-calorie/dieting phase in this program. This dieting phase in reality, serves two very important purposes. First, we want to strip off what fat will be acquired during the two-week bulking phase. This is very significant, as bodybuilders want to gain muscle, not fat.

A second very important aspect of the dieting phase

of this program is to "reprime" your body's enzymes and anabolic hormones. By alternating these two phases, the levels are maintained a constant level because you are literally tricking your own body into storing more calories as muscle tissue after a deficit.

 The great thing about these short, low-calorie, one-week dieting phases is that you begin your body's "momentum" of fat loss during this time, and it will require time to reverse the momentum towards gaining mass during the next bulking cycle.

So how many calories should somebody eat on the bulking phase and cutting program? A rough guideline-a place to start-would be to take your bodyweight times 12 [to approximate maintenance-calorie intake for an individual who's not extremely active] and add 1,500 calories to this number. For example, a person who weighs 200 lbs., like yourself, would consume about 4,000 calories a day during the bulking phase [200 x 12 = 2,400 + 1,500]. On the low-calorie phase, I would advocate consuming a number of calories equal to your bodyweight times eight. That would be about 1,600 calories for you [200 x 8 = 1,600].

 This is just a rough place to start-a person's activity level [whether they have desk jobs or are construction workers could make a big difference] and a person's muscle mass and metabolism also come into play. If a bodybuilder is abiding by this recommendation and not gaining weight during a bulking phase, I would recommend increasing calorie intake by 500 calories a day, for a week, and if a substantial weight gain is not realized, I would take it up 500 more calories the next week.

 Likewise, if someone is not losing bodyweight on the

low-calorie phase, I would recommend decreasing calorie intake by 300 calories a day, per week. Remember that each time you start an anabolic phase, you may need to increase your calorie intake, provided you're gaining lean body mass. For example, if you go from 190 to 195 lbs. during your first anabolic and fat-burning cycle, you should add about 100 more calories to your diet per day for the next cycle.

If you don't gain a significant amount of weight on the bulking phase or lose weight during each dieting phase, I would highly advocate that all those who try this system keep track of their calories as best they can, simply by writing down what they eat each day, the time they eat it, and do their best to calculate how many calories they're consuming-this data could be recorded in a notebook or journal. Having a record of what you've done will allow you to troubleshoot your program very effectively. If you're not gaining a significant amount of weight [at least three pounds a week during the bulking phase], then you need to increase your calorie intake. During the cutting phase, if you don't lose weight, you need to consume less calories. It's very simple to make adjustments on this program.

In addition to keeping a journal, it would also be very beneficial to keep track of your body composition and actually maintain an updated line graph to gauge your progress.
This is the type of bodybuilding program I would highly recommend to drug-free weight trainers who are trying to increase muscle mass without gaining fat. On this program, it's even possible to lose bodyfat while you gain muscle mass, but I would not recommend it for the obese.

I'm not sure this program would work for someone who's using steroids or who has just completed a steroid cycle. I'm concerned that if someone is coming off a steroid cycle, the body's endocrine system may not function properly and will not respond to the anabolic stimulus of a hypercaloric diet. I would have the same concern about someone who is presently using steroids-the body may not respond optimally because of all the interrupted feedback loops.

Here is a side note to what I've been saying, and something I've even considered. If you try to create your own "super-enhanced" bulking and fat-burning cycles by taking insulin, growth hormone, and fast-acting oral steroids for two weeks while consuming a lot of calories and then went on fat-burning drugs, like Cytomel and clenbuterol, and consumed a low-calorie diet for two weeks, you will actually blunt its own production of the hormones, increase the breakdown and excretion, decrease receptor sensitivity and number, increase the amount of binding proteins, and so on. While in the latter case, the body has created a hormonal environment aimed for anabolism and will not counteract itself. This way, the cycle will work very well every time you try it. I actually can't see any advantages to using drugs during this program.

If you are already consuming an excess number of calories, you should start the program with the low-calorie phase to "reprime" their anabolic systems, so to speak.

If are already on a low-calorie diet, let's say they're getting ready for a bodybuilding contest or a photo shoot, following this would be an excellent time to start the program with a high-calorie phase. In fact, many bodybuilders will probably recognize that they have "unintentionally" done a high-calorie dieting phase already-anyone who's cut up for a contest and then "pigged out" for a few weeks afterwards will confirm he/she gained size and strength at a phenomenal rate, and not all of the weight gained was fat. Ask them-they'll confirm this!

One of the things that's often discussed in bodybuilding is that those who compete make better gains, year in and year out, than those who don't because they're forced to go on calorie cycles, albeit rather traditional, longer ones. My acute, one-week calorie cycles will produce even better results than competitive bodybuilders get from cutting up and bulking up. On this system, you're literally bulking and cutting every month.

Traditionally, high-calorie diets are associated with several undesirable effects, such as increased cholesterol levels and a greater risk of cardiovascular disease, but since the overfeeding phases are only one week in length and are followed by a fat-loss phase, I don't believe there will be any adverse health consequences. I think the program is very safe and, the program has numerous advantages over other diets, which make it much easier to follow, henceforth more effective, such as: it offers variation, thus it won't become tedious to follow; it doesn't induce a mental state where you can't function within a social context; it's based on legitimate scientific findings; the "perfect" ratio of macronutrients in every meal is relatively insignificant; overall, the diet is relatively easy to follow; and the program allows you to make changes within the framework of the diet in regards to your personal ambitions and goals.

All of these things that I just brought up are not true of ketogenic diets, the Zone Diet, very high-protein diets, starvation diets, very low-fat diets, high-carbohydrate diets, and high-fat diets.

In Conclusion, you actually do have access to some powerful anabolic hormones-the good stuff! You really do have a source for actual insulin, IGF-1, and testosterone-a source you can use to pack on pounds of new muscle! And, now you know some things about how to tap into that source and how to use your body's natural biochemistry to build muscle size and strength faster than you might have ever imagined!

There are two phases of training in the following plan. Phase I is a high rep/lower calorie phase. Phase II is the low rep/high calorie phase.

Prior to the weight training portion, on any given day, warm-up on either the treadmill, stationary bike, elliptical machine or stair climber for 10 minutes.

On the high repetition/cutting phase, do about 30 min. of additional cardio, after completion of weight training.

TRAINING

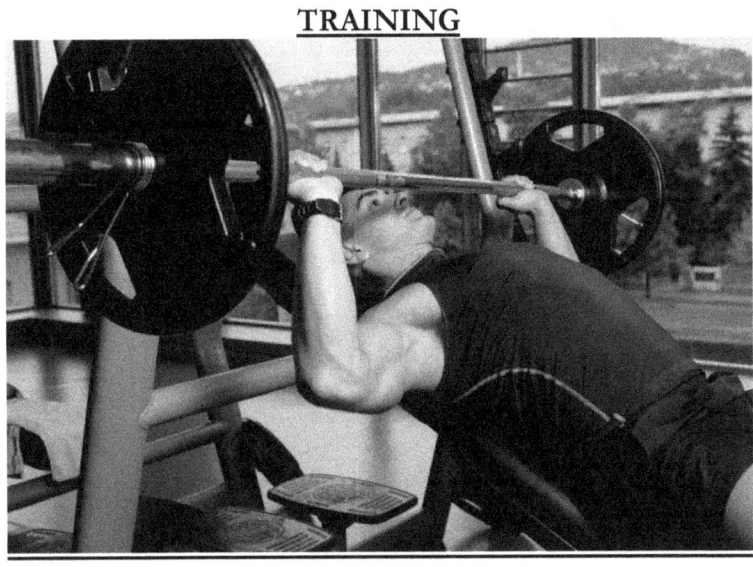

PHASE I: WEEK 1
Rest-pause set as the last set of each exercise

WORKOUT 1: HEAVY PUSH

EXERCISE	SETS/REPS
Bench Press w/Bar	4x6
Incline Bench Press w/ Bar	4x6
Incline Dumbbell Flye	4x6
Cable Crossovers (Low to High)	4x6
Military Press with Bar	4x6
Lateral Dumbbell Raises	4x6
Front Dumbbell Raises	4x6
Seated Overhead Tricep Extension	4x6
Dips	4x6

WORKOUT 2: HEAVY PULL

EXERCISE	SETS/REPS
Seated Cable Wide High Row	4x6
Chin Up/Palms in	4x6
Lat Pulldown	4x6
Seated Cable Low Row	4x8
Dumbbell Shrugs	4x8
Rear Delt Flye	4x8
Barbell Curl	4x10
Alternating Single Arm Preacher	4x10
Alternating Single Arm Cable Curl	4x10

WORKOUT 3: HEAVY LEGS

EXERCISE	SETS/REPS
Barbell Squat	4x6
Hack Squat	4x6
Leg Press	4x8
Stiff-leg Deadlift	4x8
Leg Extension	4x8
Leg Curl	4x8
Standing Calf Raise	4x8
Seated Calf Raise	4x8
Decline Sit-up	4x10
Hanging Leg Raise	4x10

PHASE I: WEEK 2
Rest-pause set as the last set of each exercise

WORKOUT 1: LIGHT PUSH

EXERCISE	SETS/REPS
Bench Press w/Dumbbells	4x12
Incline Bench Press with Bar	4x12
Incline Dumbbell Flye	4x12
Cable Crossovers (Low to High)	4x12
Military Press with Dumbbells	4x12
Lateral Cable Raises	4x12
Front Cable Raises	4x12
Seated Overhead Tricep Extension	4x12
Triceps Pushdown	4x12

WORKOUT 2: LIGHT PULL

EXERCISE	SETS/REPS
Wide-grip Lat Pulldown	4x12
Palms-In Pulldown	4x12
Dumbbell Single-Arm Row	4x12
Upright Row	4x12
Dumbbell Shrug	4x12
Rear Delt Flye	4x12
Straight Bar Arm Curl	4x12
Biceps Preacher Curl	4x12
Seated Alternating Dumbbell Curl	4x12

WORKOUT 3: LIGHT LEGS

EXERCISE	SETS/REPS
Barbell Squat	4x12
Step-Ups w/Dumbbells	4x12
Smith Machine Lunge	4x12
Leg Press	4x12
Leg Extension	4x12
Leg Curl	4x12
Rope Ab Crunch	4x12
Decline Ab Crunch	4x12

Phase II: Week 3
If you can do more than 6 repetitions, increase the weight until only 6 reps can be done. The cadence for the single sets are 10 seconds up (contraction), and 5 seconds down (negative).

Rest-pause set as the last set of each exercise

WORKOUT 1: HEAVY PUSH

EXERCISE	SETS/REPS
Bench Press w/Bar	4x6
Incline Bench Press w/ Bar	4x6
Incline Dumbbell Flye	4x6
Cable Crossovers (Low to High)	4x6
Military Press with Bar	4x6
Lateral Dumbbell Raises	4x6
Front Dumbbell Raises	4x6
Seated Overhead Tricep Extension	4x6
Dips	4x6

WORKOUT 2: HEAVY PULL

EXERCISE	SETS/REPS
Seated Cable Wide High Row	4x6
Chin Up/Palms in	4x6
Lat Pulldown	4x6
Seated Cable Low Row	4x8
Dumbbell Shrugs	4x8
Rear Delt Flye	4x8
Barbell Curl	4x10
Alternating Single Arm Preacher	4x10
Alternating Single Arm Cable Curl	4x10

WORKOUT 3: HEAVY LEGS

EXERCISE	SETS/REPS
Barbell Squat	4x6
Hack Squat	4x6
Leg Press	4x8
Stiff-leg Deadlift	4x8
Leg Extension	4x8
Leg Curl	4x8
Standing Calf Raise	4x8
Seated Calf Raise	4x8
Decline Sit-up	4x10
Hanging Leg Raise	4x10

Phase II: Week 4

If you can do more than 12 repetitions, increase the weight until only 12 reps can be done. The cadence for the single sets is rapid.

WORKOUT 1: LIGHT PUSH

EXERCISE	SETS/REPS
Bench Press w/Dumbbells	4x12
Incline Bench Press with Bar	4x12
Incline Dumbbell Flye	4x12
Cable Crossovers (Low to High)	4x12
Military Press with Dumbbells	4x12
Lateral Cable Raises	4x12
Front Cable Raises	4x12
Seated Overhead Tricep Extension	4x12
Triceps Pushdown	4x12

WORKOUT 2: LIGHT PULL

EXERCISE	SETS/REPS
Wide-grip Lat Pulldown	4x12
Palms-In Pulldown	4x12
Dumbbell Single-Arm Row	4x12
Upright Row	4x12
Dumbbell Shrug	4x12
Rear Delt Flye	4x12
Straight Bar Arm Curl	4x12
Biceps Preacher Curl	4x12
Seated Alternating Dumbbell Curl	4x12

WORKOUT 3: LIGHT LEGS

EXERCISE	SETS/REPS
Barbell Squat	4x12
Step-Ups w/Dumbbells	4x12

Smith Machine Lunge	4x12
Leg Press	4x12
Leg Extension	4x12
Leg Curl	4x12
Rope Ab Crunch	4x12
Decline Ab Crunch	4x12

PHASE III: WEEK 5
Rest-pause set as the last set of each exercise

WORKOUT 1: HEAVY PUSH

EXERCISE	SETS/REPS
Bench Press w/Bar	4x6
Incline Bench Press w/ Bar	4x6
Incline Dumbbell Flye	4x6
Cable Crossovers (Low to High)	4x6
Military Press with Bar	4x6
Lateral Dumbbell Raises	4x6
Front Dumbbell Raises	4x6
Seated Overhead Tricep Extension	4x6
Dips	4x6

WORKOUT 2: HEAVY PULL

EXERCISE	SETS/REPS
Seated Cable Wide High Row	4x6
Chin Up/Palms in	4x6
Lat Pulldown	4x6
Seated Cable Low Row	4x8
Dumbbell Shrugs	4x8
Rear Delt Flye	4x8

Barbell Curl	4x10
Alternating Single Arm Preacher	4x10
Alternating Single Arm Cable Curl	4x10

WORKOUT 3: HEAVY LEGS

EXERCISE	SETS/REPS
Barbell Squat	4x6
Hack Squat	4x6
Leg Press	4x8
Stiff-leg Deadlift	4x8
Leg Extension	4x8
Leg Curl	4x8
Standing Calf Raise	4x8
Seated Calf Raise	4x8
Decline Sit-up	4x10
Hanging Leg Raise	4x10

PHASE III: WEEK 6

WORKOUT 1: LIGHT PUSH

EXERCISE	SETS/REPS
Bench Press w/Dumbbells	4x12
Incline Bench Press with Bar	4x12
Incline Dumbbell Flye	4x12
Cable Crossovers (Low to High)	4x12
Military Press with Dumbbells	4x12
Lateral Cable Raises	4x12
Front Cable Raises	4x12
Seated Overhead Tricep Extension	4x12
Triceps Pushdown	4x12

WORKOUT 2: LIGHT PULL

EXERCISE	SETS/REPS
Wide-grip Lat Pulldown	4x12
Palms-In Pulldown	4x12
Dumbbell Single-Arm Row	4x12
Upright Row	4x12
Dumbbell Shrug	4x12
Rear Delt Flye	4x12
Straight Bar Arm Curl	4x12
Biceps Preacher Curl	4x12
Seated Alternating Dumbbell Curl	4x12

WORKOUT 3: LIGHT LEGS

EXERCISE	SETS/REPS
Barbell Squat	4x12
Step-Ups w/Dumbbells	4x12
Smith Machine Lunge	4x12
Leg Press	4x12
Leg Extension	4x12
Leg Curl	4x12
Rope Ab Crunch	4x12
Decline Ab Crunch	4x12

Phase IV: WEEK 7
Rest-pause set as the last set of each exercise

WORKOUT 1: HEAVY PUSH

EXERCISE	SETS/REPS

Exercise	Sets/Reps
Bench Press w/Bar	4x6
Incline Bench Press w/ Bar	4x6
Incline Dumbbell Flye	4x6
Cable Crossovers (Low to High)	4x6
Military Press with Bar	4x6
Lateral Dumbbell Raises	4x6
Front Dumbbell Raises	4x6
Seated Overhead Tricep Extension	4x6
Dips	4x6

WORKOUT 2: HEAVY PULL

EXERCISE	SETS/REPS
Seated Cable Wide High Row	4x6
Chin Up/Palms in	4x6
Lat Pulldown	4x6
Seated Cable Low Row	4x8
Dumbbell Shrugs	4x8
Rear Delt Flye	4x8
Barbell Curl	4x10
Alternating Single Arm Preacher	4x10
Alternating Single Arm Cable Curl	4x10

WORKOUT 3: HEAVY LEGS

EXERCISE	SETS/REPS
Barbell Squat	4x6
Hack Squat	4x6
Leg Press	4x8
Stiff-leg Deadlift	4x8
Leg Extension	4x8
Leg Curl	4x8
Standing Calf Raise	4x8

Seated Calf Raise	4x8
Decline Sit-up	4x10
Hanging Leg Raise	4x10

PHASE IV: WEEK 8
Rest-pause set as the last set of each exercise

WORKOUT 1: LIGHT PUSH

EXERCISE	SETS/REPS
Bench Press w/Dumbbells	4x12
Incline Bench Press with Bar	4x12
Incline Dumbbell Flye	4x12
Cable Crossovers (Low to High)	4x12
Military Press with Dumbbells	4x12
Lateral Cable Raises	4x12
Front Cable Raises	4x12
Seated Overhead Tricep Extension	4x12
Triceps Pushdown	4x12

WORKOUT 2: LIGHT PULL

EXERCISE	SETS/REPS
Wide-grip Lat Pulldown	4x12
Palms-In Pulldown	4x12
Dumbbell Single-Arm Row	4x12
Upright Row	4x12
Dumbbell Shrug	4x12
Rear Delt Flye	4x12
Straight Bar Arm Curl	4x12
Biceps Preacher Curl	4x12
Seated Alternating Dumbbell Curl	4x12

WORKOUT 3: LIGHT LEGS

EXERCISE	SETS/REPS
Barbell Squat	4x12
Step-Ups w/Dumbbells	4x12
Smith Machine Lunge	4x12
Leg Press	4x12
Leg Extension	4x12
Leg Curl	4x12
Rope Ab Crunch	4x12
Decline Ab Crunch	4x12

PHASE V: WEEK 9
Rest-pause set as the last set of each exercise

WORKOUT 1: HEAVY PUSH

EXERCISE	SETS/REPS
Bench Press w/Bar	4x6
Incline Bench Press w/ Bar	4x6
Incline Dumbbell Flye	4x6
Cable Crossovers (Low to High)	4x6
Military Press with Bar	4x6
Lateral Dumbbell Raises	4x6
Front Dumbbell Raises	4x6
Seated Overhead Tricep Extension	4x6
Dips	4x6

WORKOUT 2: HEAVY PULL

EXERCISE	SETS/REPS
Seated Cable Wide High Row	4x6
Chin Up/Palms in	4x6
Lat Pulldown	4x6
Seated Cable Low Row	4x8
Dumbbell Shrugs	4x8
Rear Delt Flye	4x8
Barbell Curl	4x10
Alternating Single Arm Preacher	4x10
Alternating Single Arm Cable Curl	4x10

WORKOUT 3: HEAVY LEGS

EXERCISE	SETS/REPS
Barbell Squat	4x6
Hack Squat	4x6
Leg Press	4x8
Stiff-leg Deadlift	4x8
Leg Extension	4x8
Leg Curl	4x8
Standing Calf Raise	4x8
Seated Calf Raise	4x8
Decline Sit-up	4x10
Hanging Leg Raise	4x10

PHASE V: WEEK 10

Rest-pause set as the last set of each exercise

WORKOUT 1: LIGHT PUSH

EXERCISE	SETS/REPS
Bench Press w/Dumbbells	4x12
Incline Bench Press with Bar	4x12
Incline Dumbbell Flye	4x12
Cable Crossovers (Low to High)	4x12
Military Press with Dumbbells	4x12
Lateral Cable Raises	4x12
Front Cable Raises	4x12
Seated Overhead Tricep Extension	4x12
Triceps Pushdown	4x12

WORKOUT 2: LIGHT PULL

EXERCISE	SETS/REPS
Wide-grip Lat Pulldown	4x12
Palms-In Pulldown	4x12
Dumbbell Single-Arm Row	4x12
Upright Row	4x12
Dumbbell Shrug	4x12
Rear Delt Flye	4x12
Straight Bar Arm Curl	4x12
Biceps Preacher Curl	4x12
Seated Alternating Dumbbell Curl	4x12

WORKOUT 3: LIGHT LEGS

EXERCISE	SETS/REPS
Barbell Squat	4x12
Step-Ups w/Dumbbells	4x12
Smith Machine Lunge	4x12
Leg Press	4x12
Leg Extension	4x12
Leg Curl	4x12
Rope Ab Crunch	4x12

Decline Ab Crunch   4x12

PHASE VI: WEEK 11

Rest-pause set as the last set of each exercise

WORKOUT 1: HEAVY PUSH

EXERCISE	SETS/REPS
Bench Press w/Bar	4x6
Incline Bench Press w/ Bar	4x6
Incline Dumbbell Flye	4x6
Cable Crossovers (Low to High)	4x6
Military Press with Bar	4x6
Lateral Dumbbell Raises	4x6
Front Dumbbell Raises	4x6
Seated Overhead Tricep Extension	4x6
Dips	4x6

WORKOUT 2: HEAVY PULL

EXERCISE	SETS/REPS
Seated Cable Wide High Row	4x6
Chin Up/Palms in	4x6
Lat Pulldown	4x6
Seated Cable Low Row	4x8
Dumbbell Shrugs	4x8
Rear Delt Flye	4x8
Barbell Curl	4x10
Alternating Single Arm Preacher	4x10
Alternating Single Arm Cable Curl	4x10

WORKOUT 3: HEAVY LEGS

EXERCISE	SETS/REPS
Barbell Squat	4x6
Hack Squat	4x6
Leg Press	4x8
Stiff-leg Deadlift	4x8
Leg Extension	4x8
Leg Curl	4x8
Standing Calf Raise	4x8
Seated Calf Raise	4x8
Decline Sit-up	4x10
Hanging Leg Raise	4x10

PHASE VI: WEEK 12
Rest-pause set as the last set of each exercise

WORKOUT 1: LIGHT PUSH

EXERCISE	SETS/REPS
Bench Press w/Dumbbells	4x12
Incline Bench Press with Bar	4x12
Incline Dumbbell Flye	4x12
Cable Crossovers (Low to High)	4x12
Military Press with Dumbbells	4x12
Lateral Cable Raises	4x12
Front Cable Raises	4x12
Seated Overhead Tricep Extension	4x12
Triceps Pushdown	4x12

WORKOUT 2: LIGHT PULL

EXERCISE	SETS/REPS
Wide-grip Lat Pulldown	4x12
Palms-In Pulldown	4x12
Dumbbell Single-Arm Row	4x12
Upright Row	4x12
Dumbbell Shrug	4x12
Rear Delt Flye	4x12
Straight Bar Arm Curl	4x12
Biceps Preacher Curl	4x12
Seated Alternating Dumbbell Curl	4x12

WORKOUT 3: LIGHT LEGS

EXERCISE	SETS/REPS
Barbell Squat	4x12
Step-Ups w/Dumbbells	4x12
Smith Machine Lunge	4x12
Leg Press	4x12
Leg Extension	4x12
Leg Curl	4x12
Rope Ab Crunch	4x12
Decline Ab Crunch	4x12

KEY POINTS TO SUCCESSFULLY GETTING BIG

BUILDING STRENGTH IS YOUR GOAL

Build strength, don't demonstrate it! A workout is one thing; a competitive weightlifting contest is a different matter. The best way to build strength has little in common with the best way to demonstrate strength. Yet many bodybuilders make the mistake of training as if they were in a weightlifting contest, perhaps being more interested in pressing their peers than trying to build muscular size and strength.

Olympic lifters and powerlifters postpractice maximum, single attempt lives, both in training and in competition. But there is no reason for bodybuilders ever to attempt heavy singles. While maximum muscular size cannot be produced without maximum muscular strength, it does not follow that building strength requires heavy single attempt lifts. On the contrary, greater strength and size will result from the performance of super slow repetitions within the 4 to 8 range.

Maximum size and strength can be produced without ever exerting maximum force, even though maximum contraction force is required for maximum growth stimulation. For growth stimulation. It is only necessary to produce momentary maximum contraction force. This can and should be done only after your momentary ability has been reduced by the performance of at least three repetitions that did not involve maximum contraction force. In effect, by the time you produce maximum force, your momentary ability will be reduced to the point at which the danger of injury is greatly decreased.

Bodybuilders do not hurt themselves during a first repetition because they were not warmed up properly. They hurt themselves because they are strongest at that point in the set, and they make the mistake of moving at maximum speed at a time when this results in more pull and much more jerk from the geometrical increase in the acceleration factor. Since single attempt lifts are always first repetitions. It should be evident that they are the most dangerous type of movements.

Since maximum growth stimulation can be used by momentary maximum contraction force, most of the potential danger can be avoided by reducing the existing level of ability before producing maximum force. Once again, you can accomplish this by performing 304 repetitions immediately prior to a maximal movement. Or it can be even better accomplished by pretty exhausting the muscles by working them in an isolated fashion immediately prior to involving them in a heavier, multi-joint movement.

PRE-EXHAUSTION

Pre-exhaustion makes it possible to work almost any large muscle harder than would normally be possible.
In exercises involving two or more muscles and joints, a point of failure is reached when the weakest muscle is no longer able to continue. In this case, little growth stimulation is provided for the stronger muscle involved in the same exercise.

The bench press, for example, failures usually reached when the triceps and deltoid muscles fatigue. This happens before the stronger pectoral muscles have been worked as hard as necessary to produce the best possible results. By pre-exhausting the pectoral muscles, the problem can be solved.
First, do the triceps extension in the super slow style for maximum repetitions. Second, do front deltoid raises in the same manner. Third, do the bench press, but allow no rest, following the triceps press down, not even for a second. Run immediately to the bench press and start benching.

You'll find that very little resistance is required for the bench press, probably less than half the amount of weight that you normally will use. Regardless of the lightweight being used, when you do reach a point of failure in your bench pressing, it will not be because your triceps or deltoids fatigue before your pectoralis major and minor for work properly. When you fail, it will be because your chest is exhausted. And your pecs will be worked out far harder than previously.
By pre-exhausting your chest before bench pressing, you have removed the weak link represented by triceps and deltoids involved in bench

pressing.

Other examples of pre-exhaustion that are applied are trunk curl, followed by hanging leg raise, back race, followed by stiff leg dead lift, and lateral raise followed by overhead press. In these cases, the single joint exercise precedes the multiple joint movements. Sometimes two or more single joint movements are stacked before the final exercise, which makes the cycle even harder.

In all cycles, however, keep the time between exercises to three seconds or less. Thus you may need to rearrange the equipment accordingly. Once you understand pre-exhaustion, you can use it to enormous advantage in almost every workout.

STRONGER PEOPLE NEED LESS

While proper exercise is capable of producing enormous increases in muscular mass and strength, it apparently does not produce a proportionate increase in the capability of your recovery ability.

In practice, this means that a stronger person literally cannot stand as much high-intensity work as a weaker person. When regular training is started a beginner will grow rapidly as a result of high-intensity training, even if he trains three or four times as much as required. Apparently a week individual is unable to exceed the recovery ability of his system. He is not strong enough to impose a demand on his recovery ability that cannot be met. As he become stronger, he starts making demands on his recovery ability that are difficult to meet. Now, his ability to make such demands is increasing more rapidly than his ability to meet them. Eventually, a level greater than average strength has been achieved, he becomes capable of making demands that simply cannot be met. At this strength level, the amount, duration and frequency of training must be reduced. The body needs to recover.

AND THE MOST DANGEROUS REPITITION IS......

Most bodybuilders believe that they are avoiding injury if they terminate a set prior to the most difficult repetitions. They consider the last repetitions the most dangerous. In fact, the opposite is true.

The farther you progress into a set, the safer the work.

Regardless of the number of repetitions involved in a set, the first repetition is the most dangerous in the last repetition is the safest. The more difficult it feels the safer it is, the more dangerous it seems the safer it is.

The last of the repetitions, for example, feels harder to do because you are the most exhausted, by the time you reach that point in the set. You do not feel your actual output; instead you feel the percentage of your momentarily possible output. If you can press 200 pounds, then 100 pounds will feel light to you during the first repetition and will feel heavier doing each following repetition. By the time you reach a point at which you are capable of performing one more repetition, the 100 pounds will feel very heavy. At that moment the hundred pounds you are lifting will actually be very heavy, since it will momentarily require 100% of your strength to move it.

Everything is relative in so far as feelings are concerned. The danger of injury, however, is not related directly to those feelings. Instead, your connective tissues have an actual level of resistance to pull, and since they do not perform work in the sense that they do not contract like muscles, their resistance is not reduced during the performance of a set of several repetitions. If a particular tendon has an existing level of resistance capable of withstanding 100 units of pull, then that level of resistance remains constant throughout a set. It will be 100 units during the first repetition and 100 units during the eighth repetition. Yet the danger factor changes. During the first repetition you might be momentarily capable of exerting 200 units of Pull. If you do so, then an injury will surely result. By the time you reach the eighth repetition, however, you're momentary ability may be reduced to only 10 units of Pull. At that point, you are not strong enough to hurt yourself.

Unfortunately, most bodybuilders avoid the most productive repetitions in all their sets because of an unjustified fear of injury. After working right up to the point at which one more repetition would have done some good, they stop. They are actually affording the safest repetition of all, the only one capable of producing the maximum growth stimulation they seek.

Don't let this happen in your training, always work through those last repetitions.

WHY ARE SUPER SLOW REPITITIONS MORE EFFECTIVE?

Believing in the super-slow style takes practice, especially since you probably have to reduce the weight initially to learn the form. Here are some reasons why super slow is more effective, and efficient than faster styles of lifting and lowering.
•   More muscle tension: slow repetitions produce a longer period of effective muscle tension. Faster repetitions employed more momentum and less tension or effort.
•   More muscle force: iso kinetic evaluations of maximum strength consistently revealed that more muscle force is generated as slower movement speeds. Because of this, fast repetitions are counterproductive for maximal strength development.
•   More muscle fibers: muscle force can be increased by activating more muscle fibers or by speeding up the firing rate. Because the firing rate at slow speeds does not exceed the firing rate at fast speeds, the greater muscle force produced at slow speeds is apparently due to greater recruitment of muscle fibers.
•   More muscle power: power is the production of force times speed. Power can be enhanced by increasing muscle force, the movement speed or both. Each component, however, must be trained separately for optimal results. Combining strength training with speed training is not an effective method for improving either this trait factor or the speed factor. You can lift heavy weights slowly or lightweights quickly. Because near maximum resistance is essential for maximum strength development, it is recommended that you train with relatively heavy weights and slow speeds to enhance the force factor. As more muscle strength is developed, the force factor increases and permits greater power production.
•   Less tissue trauma: slow lifting movements accomplish the same amount of work and produce greater muscle tension that fast lifting movements, but slow weight training causes less tissue trauma at the start and finish of the exercise movements and is less likely to cause injuries. Slow repetitions should be the preferred technique for

building muscle.

• Less momentum: momentum plays a part in virtually all forms of exercise, the faster the movement, the greater the momentum. This is an important consideration, because as the momentum component increases, the muscle component decreases momentum assisted exercises give the appearance of greater muscle strength, but actually decreases demand on the target muscle groups and increases stress on joints.

THE KEY TO PROPER BREATHING

One of the real challenges in using super slow, especially when going heavier is the more intense work is done, the more you feel you're not getting enough air. You're probably holding your breath, taking a deep breath, holding your breath, taking a deep breath, and so on. In other words, you are off and on breathing.

Many times such breathing is synced to jerking or moving the weight too fast. Actually, what is desired is the exact opposite: spaced continuous, relax, ventilation, combined with a steady contraction force.

Try not to hold your breath while doing any super slow repetition. Keep your mouth open, relax your face and neck, and breath.

Deep breaths are not necessary. In fact, it's your benefit to practice short, rapid breaths with emphasis on blowing out rather than taking in large gulps of air. Try to ventilate just enough so your breathing never stops.

Doing so will reduce the tendency that you may have to get dizzy or develop a headache. It will also increase the load of the muscle, which will lead to greater growth stimulation.

Emphasize short, rapid breathing in and out during your training session today and see if it doesn't lead to performance of at least one more repetition in each exercise.

RECOVERY

On an off day, you should be getting lots of rest and lots of food and drink. After days of training, you need to concentrate on replenishing your recovering abilities.

Recovery ability is defined as a chemical reactions that are necessary for your body to produce muscular growth. Optimal recovery ability is dependent on adequate rest, talents, nutrition and time.

Muscular size and strength occur ordinarily as part of normal growth. As a bodybuilder, however, you seek abnormal levels. Your objective is to build maximum levels of muscular size from shortest amount of time, from the least amount of effort. It only follows that you should be looking for the most productive method of exercise.

A healthy body will provide normal levels of size and strength. According to its perception of what is needed for normal requirements, plus a bit more, as reserved for emergency use. As long as existing levels are adequate, as long as extreme demands are not made on the body, no additional size or strength will be provided. To produce growth, demands must be made in excess of normal. Only then will the body attempt to provide the size and strength required to meet these demands. If it can.

Your body is a complex factory, constantly making hundreds of delicate changes that transform food and oxygen into many chemicals needed by various parts of the system. But there is a limit to the chemical conversions that your recovery ability can make within a given time. If your requirements exceed that limit, your body will eventually be overworked to the point of collapse.

The recovery ability of your body provides normal growth. It also provides abnormal growth, if such abnormal growth is dictated, and if the recovery ability is able to meet the requirements. It is not possible for you to exhaust your recovery ability while doing nothing to stimulate abnormal growth. Obviously, then, to be productive, and exercise must stimulate abnormal growth as much as possible while disturbing the recovery ability as little as possible. Under this concept an ideal exercise would be infinitely hard and infinitely brief. It will provide maximum growth stimulation while leaving your recovery ability in the best possible shape to meet the requirements for growth.

Take advantage of your off day and the subsequent off days as they occur on a more frequent basis. The right amount of rest, relaxation, and time are necessary for getting bigger.

NUTRITION

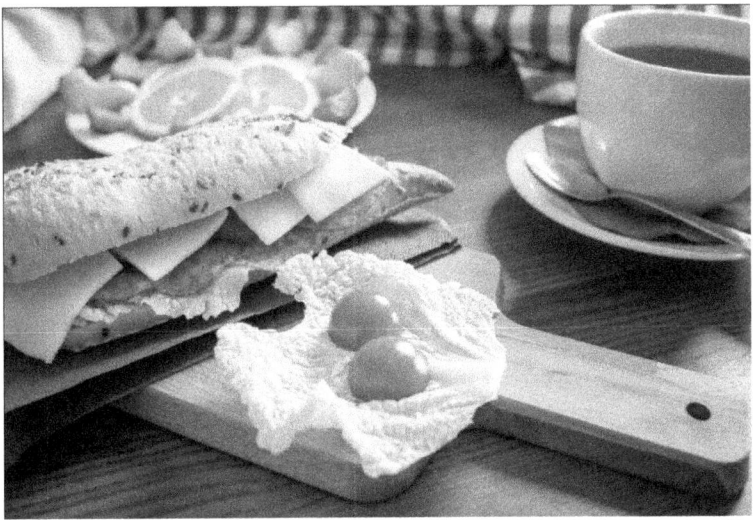

The Bulking Phase

Start this system by consuming 1,500 more calories per day more than your maintenance energy requirements. If you're not very active, and basically sit behind a desk all day and then work out for an hour, you probably burn fewer calories each day than those of you who take part in a lot of recreational sports, have physically demanding jobs, etc. Anyway, for some, 2,400-2,800 calories a day is their maintenance intake. So, consume around 4,000-4,200 calories per day to start with. If you don't put on at least three pounds the first week, go up to about 4,700 calories a day the second week. The plan is to consume 6 meals every day, each with about 500 to 800 calories.

Protein, Carbs, and Fat:

In the bulking phase, a 20% protein, 50% carb, and 30% fat macronutrient profile will work well. You can go with a bit more protein, but an emphasis must be on a relatively high level of carbs consumed while bulking. That will maximize insulin output and help promote anabolism.

An example of the bulking phase diet:

4000 Calorie Meal 1	Calories	Protein	Carbs	Fat
4 Whole Eggs	320	28	0	20
4 Egg Whites	80	15	0	0
Bagel	210	8	42	2
Cream Cheese	50	1	0	5
Totals	660	52	42	27

4000 Calorie Meal 2	Calories	Protein	Carbs	Fat
Protein Powder – 2 scoops	240	44	8	4

	Calories	Protein	Carbs	Fat
Skim Milk – 12 ounces	120	12	16	0
Banana	121	1	31	0
Natural Peanut Butter – 1 tablespoon	97	4	3	9
Oatmeal	100	4	19	2
Totals	678	65	77	15

4000 Calorie Meal 3	Calories	Protein	Carbs	Fat
Top Sirloin Steak – 10 ounces	650	108	0	20
Brown Rice – 1 serving	220	6	40	4
Sweet Potato	103	2	24	0
Totals	973	116	64	24

4000 Calorie Meal 4	Calories	Protein	Carbs	Fat
Protein Powder – 2 scoops	240	44	8	4
Skim Milk – 12 ounces	120	12	16	0
Banana	121	1	31	0
Peanut Butter – 1 teaspoon	97	4	3	9
Totals	578	61	58	13

4000 Calorie Meal 5	Calories	Protein	Carbs	Fat
Grilled Salmon – 8 ounces	464	48	0	24
Brown Rice – 1 serving	220	6	40	4
Veggies/Small Salad	50	1	10	1
Totals	734	55	50	29

4000 Calorie Meal 6	Calories	Protein	Carbs	Fat
Protein Powder – 2 scoops	240	44	8	4
Skim Milk – 12 ounces	120	12	16	0
Natural Peanut Butter – 1 tablespoon	97	4	3	9
Totals	457	60	27	13

	Calories	Protein	Carbs	Fat
Totals	4080	409	318	121

If you have a problem eating every few hours, a blender can become your best friend. You can whip up a blender Power Shake, and drink it down, filling your system with plenty of nutrients, without taking a lot of your time. Here's an example of an inexpensive blender drink that I often use:

8 ounces of yogurt (any flavor), low fat or not, it's your choice
1 medium banana
1 cup of milk (2%)
Ice cubes (optional)

Water to thin (if necessary)

This Shake delivers to your body 488 calories, 80 grams of carbohydrates, 24 grams of protein, and 8 grams of fat.
(If you're a hard gainer like me, you'll add some protein powder, and maybe even a few cookies.)

The Cutting Phase

After two weeks of overfeeding during the bulking cycle, you need to "shift gears" and go on a low-calorie diet. Because you'll be trying to lose fat at a very rapid pace during this two-week cutting period, you'll need to create a significant energy deficit. You have to go down to around 1,600-1,800 calories a day for 14 days in order to accomplish my objective. Basically, you're going to starve your butt off. Plan to eat small meals often throughout the day.

Protein, Carbs, and Fat:

During the cutting phase, reduce your carbohydrate intake substantially. You'll be consuming a diet that will be around 40-45% protein, 40-45% carbs, and 10-20% fat.

An example of what an average day's food intake might be on the low-calorie phase is shown below.

Example of a Daily Nutrition Program during the Cutting Phase. Any of the foods can be substituted with a food from the same food group.

Breakfast

1 Cup 1% Milk
1 Banana, small
Maple-Nut Granola

Morning Snack
2 Whole-Grain Rice Cake
1 Peach, medium

Lunch
Tex-Mex Taco Salad
1 Cup 1% Milk
1 Corn Tortilla
1/2 Cup Nonfat Strawberry Frozen Yogurt

Afternoon Snack
1 Ounce Pistachios, unsalted

Dinner
3/4 Cup Cooked Couscous
3/4 Cup Mashed Acorn Squash
Tuscan Pork Loin
1 Cup Strawberries

Additional Tips and Tricks

During the bulking phase:
1. Always eat something for breakfast.
2. 1 teaspoon of honey in 1 cup of milk, in the morning, on an empty stomach.
3. 2-3 bananas +1 glass of milk immediately following increases weight very fast.
4. 10 raisins before going to bed, then drink fresh water, then go to sleep. This corrects metabolism, and increases weight fast.

During the cutting phase, just stick to some basic rules:

1. No fruit and juices after breakfast. Juices, even fruit juices, contain a lot of sugar, which triggers higher insulin levels in your blood, which causes the body to store fat.

2. No pasta, rice, bread, or potatoes after 6 pm. Complex carbs take more time for the body to break down, unlike simple sugars.

3. Eat more meat (chicken breast), and up the amount of vegetables you consume. Vegetables contain sugar in the form of cellulose. The human body cannot digest cellulose, therefore we pass it straight throughout bodies (vegetables look the same coming out as they did going in). Only cows and goats have the machinery to digest cellulose.

4. Make sure you're drinking plenty of water, about 2 L/day (8 x 8oz.)

5. Increase your cardio time at the end of your workout. (Treadmill, Elliptical trainer, etc.)

Stick to this routine and the results will astonish you. Without a doubt you'll be blown away by the results on the scale, and in the mirror.

ABOUT THE AUTHOR

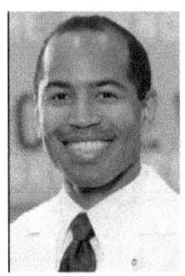

Dr. R. Conrad Bingham, D.D.S., NASM-CPT,
has competed in natural amateur bodybuilding contest on the east
coast and in Arizona, from 1999 until 2006 as a bantam weight, light
weight, and middle weight competitor, and always placed at or near the
top of his weight classes.
In 2014, Dr. Bingham became a Certified Personal Trainer with the
National Academy of Sports Medicine.
Dr. Bingham feels that the combination of training in biology, anatomy
and physiology and the experience learned from amateur, natural
bodybuilding, and dieting, has proven to be an asset in building and
sculpting a "Championship" quality body.

www.ingramcontent.com/pod-product-compliance
Lightning Source LLC
Chambersburg PA
CBHW070819290526
45795CB00002B/766